Diabetes

The Diabetes Management Guide To Prevent, Control And Treat Diabetes Successfully

By

Richard Hall

2nd Edition

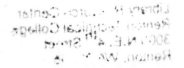

Table of Contents

Introduction

Diabetes is a common disease that afflicts more and more people every day. No wonder, since everyone is surrounded with so many tempting yet incredibly unhealthy food items, full of empty calories that prove to be too much for their bodies to bear. In addition to that, most people live a sedentary lifestyle that greatly lacks exercise and activities that are supposed to burn off any extra calories naturally. Diabetes can also be due to genetic factors, which makes it a challenging disease to avoid. In fact, despite your best efforts you may find yourself with a diagnosis of diabetes.

This book contains information that will help you understand how diabetes works, along with scientifically proven ways to treat and manage it. Look at diabetes as a wake-up call to taking better care of your body, and realize that by following these tips, you will be able to live a healthier and more productive lifestyle, despite your diabetes.

CHAPTER 1

Understanding How Diabetes Works

Diabetes is gradually becoming one of the most common health issues, affecting over 20 million people in the United States alone. One of the most important steps that you need to take in order to fight against diabetes is to understand how it works. In order to get a grasp of the roots of diabetes, you need to take a look at what happens inside the human body.

Blood Glucose

Glucose is a simple sugar that is used as an energy source by every cell in the human body. It is delivered through the bloodstream to the cells, and is then broken down to be used as energy to allow the body to function normally and healthily.

Blood glucose is obtained from food. After eating any sort of food, the glucose is taken in by the intestines and transferred to the bloodstream. The body ensures that it has an incessant supply of glucose by regulating a consistent level of it in the blood. However, when there is too much glucose, the body turns it into long chains called glycogen, and stores it in the muscles and the liver. Whenever the cells do not have enough glucose, the brain signals you to eat or else it will make use of the stored glycogen.

Insulin and Glucagon

In order for the body to preserve a consistent level of blood glucose it utilizes the hormones insulin and glucagon. Both hormones have inverse effects on the tissues that are responsible for regulating the blood glucose level.

The constant normal blood glucose concentration should stay at approximately 90 mg per 100 ml of blood.

Insulin is a protein hormone that carries 51 amino acids and it is needed by the majority of the body's cells, particularly the liver, fat cells and muscle cells. It is created and released by the beta cells of the pancreatic islets. Insulin is responsible for stimulating the liver and muscle cells to store glycogen and to produce proteins from amino acids, for triggering the fat cells to produce fats from fatty acids and glycerol, and for preventing the liver and the kidney cells from forming glucose from non-carbohydrates, a process called gluconeogenesis. Insulin, therefore, stores nutrients immediately after you have eaten by minimizing the concentrations of glucose, amino acids, and fatty acids in the bloodstream.

Whenever you are not eating, the pancreas will secrete glucagon in order for the body to produce glucose. Glucagon is also a protein hormone, but it is created and released by the alpha cells of the pancreatic islets. It is responsible for stimulating the liver and muscle cells to break down the stored glycogen for distribution to the cells, it triggers the liver and kidneys to perform gluconeogenesis, and it circulates the glucose to increase the concentrations in the bloodstream to be used as an energy source.

There is usually a healthy counter-balance of insulin and glucagon in the bloodstream. For instance, after you have eaten, they body will absorb the glucose, amino acids and fatty acids from the food in the intestine. The moment this happens, the pancreatic beta cells are triggered to secrete insulin into the blood and suppress the pancreatic alpha cells from releasing glucagon. The insulin levels will gradually increase in the blood and work on the cells to take in the glucose, amino acids and fatty acids. This function precludes the blood glucose concentration from becoming too high in the bloodstream and ensures a balance.

On the other hand, during times of fasting — which is basically the times when you are not eating — the body still requires a constant supply of glucose to survive, and this time it takes it from the blood. When the body identifies a small decrease in blood sugar levels, it stimulates the pancreatic alpha cells to release glucagon and prevent the release of insulin. This increases the blood-glucagon levels and works on the liver, kidneys and muscles to move the glucose from glycogen or to produce glucose that is secreted into the bloodstream, preventing a dangerous drop in the blood-glucose concentration.

The 3 Types of Diabetes

There are 3 types of diabetes: Type 1, Type 2, and Gestational Diabetes.

Type 1, which is also referred to as insulin-dependent diabetes or juvenile diabetes, is caused by an insufficient supply of insulin. This is because the beta cells of the pancreatic islets are destroyed, possibly due to genetics, environmental factors, or the immune system. About 5 – 10% of diabetics have Type 1 diabetes, and most of them are children and teenagers. They do not have insulin in the blood, and have an abnormal glucose tolerance.

Type 2, also referred to as adult-onset diabetes or non-insulin-dependent diabetes, takes place when the body is unable to react to or utilize its own insulin. This is a state known as insulin resistance. About 90 – 95% of diabetics have Type 2 diabetes, and the majority are adults more than 40 years old. They also have an abnormal glucose tolerance level, and have unnaturally high levels of insulin in the blood. Insulin resistance is directly associated with obesity, although more research needs to be conducted in order to better understand this link. There are some findings which suggest that the amount of insulin receptors in the muscle, liver and fat cells are reduced, while other findings suggest that there may be alterations in the intracellular pathways triggered by insulin in these cells.

Gestational diabetes almost always occurs in pregnant women, and is often likened to Type 2 diabetes. This is also evidenced by abnormal glucose tolerance, and somewhat higher insulin levels. During gestation, the effects of insulin are partially obstructed by various hormones, causing a decrease in sensitivity towards insulin. Diabetes thus develops, but is manageable by diet, together with supplemental insulin injections. Gestational diabetes usually disappears after parturition.

Understanding the Causes of Type 2 Diabetes

Genetics play a role in the development of Type 2 diabetes. For instance, research shows that when one identical twin has Type 2 diabetes, the chances of the other identical twin developing it are between 75% and 90%.

Impaired glucose tolerance – also known as pre-diabetes - takes place prior to the development of Type 2 diabetes, since the blood glucose levels are lower than normal, forcing the body to generate extra insulin in order to regulate it. A sedentary lifestyle paired with aging will further trigger the development of Type 2 diabetes, because the pancreas will be unable to keep up with the insulin demands. Another cause is the release of sugar from the liver, also referred to as hepatic glucose output. This is triggered by the abnormal release of glucose from the liver during fasting.

Contrary to popular belief, bingeing on sugary foods does not lead to Type 2 diabetes, although it will contribute to its development, since it inevitably leads to obesity. In fact, eating too much fat and protein has more or less the same effect on the body as bingeing on sugary foods.

Symptoms of Diabetes

There are a number symptoms related to diabetes, but these symptoms may also be caused by other conditions, so if you suspect you may have diabetes, you need to get checked out by your doctor as soon as possible. The most common

Symptoms of type 2 diabetes are: polydipsia or abnormal thirst, polyuria or frequent urination, extreme hunger, excessive fatigue, numbness in the hands and feet, changes in vision, unnatural weight loss, abnormally slow healing of wounds and sores, and unnatural frequency of infection.

The absence of insulin, or insulin ineffectiveness, is responsible for the symptoms mentioned above, since this prevents the cells from taking in glucose from the bloodstream, thus leading to high glucose levels in the blood. However, because the cells are unable to absorb the glucose, the body receives a message to feel hungry, which in turn causes glucagon levels rise. Glucagon then works on the muscles and liver to take apart the stored glycogen and secrete the glucose into the blood, causing the blood glucose levels to rise even more. These levels are by now so high that it cannot all be filtered by the kidneys, and this causes glucose to be excreted in the urine. It also causes people to urinate more frequently than normal. Abnormally frequent urination results in the loss of sodium from the body and causes sufferers to feel thirsty all the time.

If you are suffering from undiagnosed diabetes, you will also experience fatigue due to the fact that the cells are unable to take in glucose. The numbness of the hands and feet, changes in vision, slow healing of wounds and frequency of infections are caused by the high levels of blood glucose, which inevitably leads to compromised blood circulation. Gangrene and blindness can occur in severe cases.

You might experience weight loss regardless of your constant eating, since the absence of or resistance to insulin directly triggers the breakdown of fats and proteins in the body. This process extends to the body producing acidic ketones in the blood, causing breathing problems and irregularities in the heart and central nervous system. This can ultimately result in a diabetic coma, although this is a worst case scenario.

Explaining the serious nature of some of the physical effects of diabetes is not meant to cause worry; however, you need to fully understand the importance of taking the necessary steps to manage, treat and ultimately overcome high blood glucose by making changes in your lifestyle along with taking certain medications.

CHAPTER 2

The Importance of Undergoing Tests

Fortunately, more and more improvements have led to the development of many products and treatments for diabetes. In order to control your blood glucose and make the necessary healthy adjustments to your lifestyle, you will need to undergo several tests.

The Blood Glucose Test

Self-monitoring is the simplest and most common means of testing your blood glucose. You will need a blood glucose meter, a blood glucose record book, a lancet device, a disposable test strip, and a cotton ball.

In the blood glucose test, the glucose in your blood will react with an enzyme that can be found on your test strip. This will produce electrons which the meter can convert into a glucose reading.

To administer this test, you will first need to wash your hands and dry them thoroughly. After that, you will prick your finger using a lancet and then drop some blood onto the test strip. This test strip is then inserted into the blood glucose meter and registers the results, often including the date and time. Write down the reading in your glucose record book to take along to your next medical consultation.

It is important that you are the only person to use your meter. Do not reuse the lancet device or the test strips. In fact, test strips that have not been used for 90 days need to be disposed of, as they cannot be relied on for accuracy.

How to Find the Right Blood Glucose Meter

It is important to find the correct blood glucose meter for you, because you will need to use solely the test strips that are from the same manufacturer. Test strips cannot be interchanged with different meters.

Most reliable meters are not that expensive nowadays, and all are fairly accurate in providing you with results. However, their accuracy can be as much as 10% different from the results you get from a laboratory.

In shopping for a blood glucose meter, check whether the manufacturer offers an instantly available and reliable customer care package, and confirm the warranty period. Also check if the results will be given in mmol/L. Check if the batteries for that meter can be bought anywhere, and are easily affordable. It is also preferable that the meter has a memory and can keep track of your results. It is even better if you can download the results to your computer. If you are pregnant, check whether the meter is meant for gestational diabetes as well. Lastly, make sure that the meter is suitable for use when you are taking other medications, for these can affect the results. If you are still unsure as to which meter you should purchase, ask your doctor for recommendations.

The Glycosylated Hemoglobin or HbA1c Test

The individual blood glucose test is effective in determining your blood glucose level at a certain point in your day, giving you an idea of what you need to do in order to make adjustments. However, it is important to know the state of your blood glucose levels over time, whether in days, weeks or months. This is when you will need the HbA1c test.

Hemoglobin is a protein that transports oxygen throughout the body and distributes it to organs that need it for all the chemical reactions that are occurring naturally all the time. Hemoglobin is contained inside red blood cells and is responsible for giving these cells color. Red blood cells survive in the bloodstream for around 60 to 90 days.

Glucose binds itself in various ways to the haemoglobin, and the sum of all the hemoglobin that is bound to the glucose is referred to as *glycohemoglobin* or *glycosylated hemoglobin*. Once the red blood cells have bound themselves to the glucose, they stay bound until they die, which is about 3 months later. As the red blood cells die, new ones are developed and once more the glucose will bind itself to the new cells. The biggest portion of total glycosylated hemoglobin is named HbA1c.

The HbA1c test will measure the level of glucose bound to the red blood cells and express it in the form of a percentage. For instance, if 7 out of every 100 red blood cells have glucose bound to them, the HbA1c report will show 7 percent. Normal HbA1c levels, or those of individuals without diabetes, are from 4 to 6 percent. Testing a diabetic's HbA1c levels can give a report of the glucose control over a period of 3 months, because that is how long the cells which they are attached to live.

Blood glucose tests will measure the amount of glucose that is circulating in the blood at the period that it was conducted, therefore their unit of measurement is unlike that of the HbA1c test. The blood glucose test will measure the millimoles of glucose for every liter of blood (mmol/L). HbA1c, on the other hand, is not an average of blood glucose levels; it reports the consistently high blood glucose levels resulting in high glycosylated red blood cells, thus resulting in increasing HbA1c. It is important for a person with Type 2 Diabetes to undergo the HbA1c test four times each year.

Closely monitoring your blood glucose levels can be highly motivating and helpful in the management of your diabetes. It will remind you to stick to your eating plan and exercise program diligently. Also, these tests will enable you to make alterations to what you are doing based on personal results, instead of just following whatever generic information you can find regarding the diabetic's lifestyle.

Each person is different, and diabetes affects each person in a different way, although there is some common ground for all diabetics. Regular testing will ensure that your lifestyle and care plan is tailored to your individual requirements. This should ensure that you can live healthily without diabetes having too many adverse effects on your body. Also, significant changes will be picked up early, and the chances of treating them successfully will be higher.

CHAPTER 3

An Overview of Diabetes Treatments

Currently, there is no cure for diabetes. Once you have a diagnosis, you have to learn to live with it. Nevertheless, it can be treated and managed by following a specific lifestyle and care plan and working with your medical team. Treating diabetes involves carefully checking and managing your blood glucose levels, eating a specially tailored diet, taking your medications correctly, and doing regular exercise.

Treatment for Type 1 Diabetes

For people with Type 1 diabetes, the absence of insulin means that insulin injections need to be administered several times every day. These are typically given during mealtimes in order to contend with the amount of glucose that is taken in after eating. Blood glucose levels need to be checked several times each day as well, in order to adjust the amount of insulin that will be injected and avoid making drastic changes in the blood glucose concentration.

A Type 1 diabetic might be able to find implantable insulin infusion pumps that will enable him to simply push a button and infuse insulin. Remember that, if you inject an excessive level of insulin, you will experience hypoglycemia, the symptoms of which are nausea and trembling. This is because the brain is not getting a healthy amount of glucose. Dangerously low levels of blood glucose can lead to a coma from insulin shock and can be deadly.

Keep in mind that you should never rely on insulin injections alone to manage and treat diabetes; you must be careful of your food choices and closely monitor the carbohydrate and fat content in your diet. You should also exercise regularly. Since Type 1 diabetes is genetic, you will have to follow this program for the rest of your life, so learn as much as you can about your condition and how it affects your body. Knowledge is power, and with full knowledge of your condition, you can live a happy, healthy life, despite diabetes.

Treatment for Type 2 Diabetes

Type 2 diabetes is easily manageable by ensuring that you are maintaining your optimal fitness level by way of regular exercise and a healthy, balanced diet. You will need to perform a blood glucose test every day or whenever you visit your doctor. Medication is necessary for those who are suffering from a more serious level of Type 2 diabetes in order to control their blood glucose.

The majority of prescription drugs for Type 2 diabetes are in the form of oral medications, and they are developed for the following purposes. Triggering the pancreas to secrete more insulin so as to lower blood glucose levels; intervening in the absorption of glucose by the intestine so as to block glucose from entering the bloodstream; stimulating insulin sensitivity; lowering glucose production by the liver; assisting in metabolizing or breakdown of glucose; providing insulin to the bloodstream via injections.

Apart from medications, diabetics can also opt for alternative treatments. Although there is no scientific research or evidence that can prove, without a doubt, the effectiveness of these treatments, there have been reports of successful results.

One common alternative treatment is acupuncture, which is often administered to relieve nerve damage caused by diabetes. Adding chromium, vanadium and magnesium to the diet is another treatment because these are said to help regulate glucose-tolerance and minimize the complications linked to diabetes. It is likely that a Type 2 diabetic will have to follow this form of treatment throughout his lifetime.

There have currently been a lot of developments that can permanently treat diabetes, and they involve pancreatic islet transplantation. The islets in the pancreas of a deceased donor are transplanted via a catheter into the liver of a diabetic recipient. Given enough time, the islet cells will bind to the new blood vessels and start to release insulin. There have been successful pancreatic islet transplantations in the past, but the biggest issue is when the recipient's body rejects the donor's tissue.

Apart from diet, exercise and medication, many diabetics have started engaging in meditation and other relaxation techniques to help regulate their hormonal levels and reduce stress.

CHAPTER 4

Eating to Treat Diabetes

The food that you introduce into your body plays a major role in the treatment of diabetes. Carefully tracking your meals will help to improve your health and manage your blood glucose. Of course, it is always best to consult a dietician who specializes in diabetes so that you can tailor a meal plan that is suitable for your individual requirements.

Many diabetics, particularly those with Type 2 diabetes, are obese, and therefore weight loss and weight management is the most important issue. Losing weight will greatly lower the risk of developing Type 2 diabetes, and also prevents diabetes from getting worse. A healthy diet that is focused on weight loss can even boost the effects of medication. Lastly, achieving your optimal fitness level will enable you to lower your blood pressure, boost your energy levels and increase your life expectancy.

It is important to consider that genetics often plays a significant role in a person's ability to lose weight, and may also govern the amount that can be lost.

Those with Type 2 diabetes generally lose less weight compared to individuals without diabetes. Knowing this information will keep you grounded and prevent you from becoming frustrated if you are not getting the results that you are hoping for.

Monitor Your Calorie Intake

A calorie is the unit of measurement of energy, and the formula of weight loss is pretty simple: the number of calories that you burn off through normal bodily functions and exercise should be more than the number of calories that you take in from food. If you eat more calories than you burn off, you will naturally gain weight.

The amount of calories that your body needs depends on a variety of factors, including your age, your sex, your size and your body composition. For instance, a pregnant or breastfeeding woman will need more calories than a man who works behind a desk 8 hours a day.

The three basic food macro nutrient food groups contain the most calories, and these are proteins, fats and carbohydrates. It is necessary to cut 3,500 calories from your diet in order to lose one pound in weight, and it's healthy to aim for a weight loss of 1 – 2 lbs per week. That means cutting back by 500 – 1,000 calories a day from the basic calories your body needs to function.

Protein

The body requires a certain amount of protein in order to build and repair tissue. Children and young adults require more protein than adults because they are still growing. You can obtain protein from various sources, such as poultry, beef, pork, seafood, eggs, dairy and dairy products, legumes including soy, and nuts.

A diabetic needs to be careful in choosing his or her sources of protein because animal proteins contain saturated fat. The rule of thumb is to choose lean protein foods that can provide you more protein and less fat and calorie content. An adult diabetic should eat not more than two medium-sized amounts of protein each day, including milk and legumes. The recommended amount of protein in your daily calorie intake should be about 10 - 20% of total calories, although you should consider that protein can satisfy hunger better than carbohydrates and fat. This is useful when you're trying to lose weight as a diabetic, since the feeling of satiety also helps to stabilise blood sugar levels.

The following options are recommended for daily lean protein intake: baked or grilled lean beef, pork, veal or lamb, legumes including lentils, crab, lobster, prawns, low-fat milk, cheese and yogurt, skinless lean chicken or turkey meat, tofu, white fish, tuna, salmon, egg, and nuts. Avoid processed meats such as sausages and salami, Cheddar, feta, blue vein cream and Camembert cheeses.

Fat

It is very important to limit your fat intake, especially if you have diabetes. The maximum amount of fat in your daily calorie intake should be 30% of total calories. Dietary fat has two main categories: saturated and unsaturated.

The 'evil' fat is saturated fat and it comes mainly from animal products. Butter, bacon, cream, cheese, and pastries contain saturated fat. Saturated fat that comes from plant sources are coconut milk and palm oil. What makes saturated fat 'evil' is basically due to its effects of increasing your blood cholesterol level. Ideally, the amount of saturated fat in your daily calorie intake should not be more than one-third of the 30% total.

Unsaturated fat comes from vegetable sources including nuts and seeds and comes in two forms: monounsaturated and polyunsaturated. Monounsaturated fat will not increase your cholesterol level and is therefore the 'good' fat. You can get monounsaturated fat from canola oil, olive oil, almonds, peanuts and avocado. Polyunsaturated fat does not raise your cholesterol level either but it will reduce your HDL or 'good' cholesterol. You can get polyunsaturated fat from soybeans, sunflowers, oily fish, and sesame oil.

You can reduce the risk of heart disease if you add essential fatty acids to your diet, particularly Omega-3. If you are unable to maintain a regular intake of two to three servings of oily fish per week, or if you have problems with the absorption of Omega-3, you may benefit from fish oil supplements. Make sure that the capsules contain both EPA or *eicosapentaenoic acid* and DHA or *docosahexaenoic acid*. The recommended daily intake of fish oil is between 1,200 mgs and 3,000 mgs per day.

Carbohydrates

Ideally, diabetics should only eat complex carbohydrates, such as whole grains and brown rice, pasta and bread, since they are more nutritious, higher in fiber and lower in fat than refined carbohydrates. Your daily intake of complex carbohydrates should be around 40% of your daily calorie intake. Fiber is not digestible, but it has a number of health benefits, including promoting a healthy digestive system and protecting against heart disease.

You can find fiber in whole foods such as grains, vegetables and fruits. Furthermore, fiber helps give you that feeling of being full and so helps to control the appetite. That's a bonus when you're trying to lose weight.

Avoid simple carbohydrates that contain too many calories and not enough nutrients, such as soft drinks, alcoholic beverages, candies, jam, biscuits, cakes and refined white sugar, rice and pasta. By avoiding these foods, you are lowering your intake of glucose, thereby decreasing your blood glucose levels significantly. In addition, most simple or refined carbohydrates tend to be processed food, and that is decidedly unhealthy, whether you are diabetic or not.

It is also advisable that you check on the glycemic index or GI of the foods you eat, because that will give you an indication of how rapidly a particular carbohydrate food is digested. Complex carbohydrates take more time to be digested, therefore the release of glucose into the bloodstream from these foods is much slower which, in turn, buys time for the pancreas to keep up with their secretion of insulin. However, that does not mean that you can eat as many complex carbohydrates as you want, because these still contain fat and may raise your blood glucose levels if eaten to excess. Make sure to control your portions by spreading carbohydrates evenly across breakfast, lunch and dinner.

Other Important Nutrients

Aside from monitoring your daily calorie intake of proteins, fats and carbohydrates, you should ensure that your diet includes sufficient vitamins and minerals, especially Vitamins A, B1 or thiamine, B2 or riboflavin, B6 or pyridoxine, pantothenic acid and biotin, B12, folic acid, Niacin, Vitamin C, D, E and K, calcium, phosphorus, magnesium, iodine, iron, sodium, chromium, chlorine, cobalt, tin, zinc and so on. These are all vital to maintaining the regular functions of the different cells in your body and helping to prevent infection.

You should also monitor your daily water intake, because it is very important to the proper absorption of nutrients. It is recommended that you drink around 2 litres of water a day – that's about 6 to 8 glasses — and more if you have been exercising or in hot climates. As a diabetic, you should avoid sugary soft drinks and minimize your intake of caffeine and alcoholic beverages. Lemon water is a good way to detoxify and add some zest into plain old boring water, and herbal tea is considered to be well accepted in the diabetic diet.

How to Plan Your Meals

Living with diabetes means that serious lifestyle adjustments must be made in order to control it. In fact, careful diabetics often turn out to be healthier than their non-diabetic friends, simply because they are more conscious of the way their bodies function, as well as paying close attention to their diet and exercise regimen.

A balanced diet should have well portioned amounts of proteins, fats and carbohydrates from preferably organic and whole foods that are also chock full of vitamins and minerals. Essentially, you should have a fixed schedule for meals, since it is not healthy to go for hours without food, as this could compromise your blood glucose levels.

For instance, breakfast might be at 7 o'clock in the morning, lunch at around 12 noon, and dinner at 7 o'clock in the evening, with healthy snacks in between. If you are feeling hungry in between your meals, then drink a full glass of water because the chances are that you are simply thirsty. If you still feel famished 20 minutes after drinking, then you can opt for a light snack such as a piece of fruit to curb your appetite until the next regular meal.

When planning for the protein in your meals, you must remember that it comprises 10 – 20% of your daily intake, which is equivalent to 2 medium-sized servings per day. That is approximately equivalent to one of the following: 150 grams (5 ounces) of fish, 30 grams (1 ounce) of nuts, half a cup of cooked legumes, 40 grams (1.5 ounces) of cheese, 90 grams (3 ounces) of chicken, beef or poultry or 2 large eggs.

As for the fats in your meals, remember that they should comprise 30% at most of your daily intake and these include creams, mayonnaise, butter, oils, and margarine. Fats are also present in most protein sources. This is approximately equivalent to one tablespoon of unsaturated fats each day. Keep in mind that you cannot avoid fats completely as your body needs the essential fatty acids. The clue is in the name! Fat is also necessary for you to properly absorb fat-soluble vitamins.

In selecting your carbohydrates, remember that they should only comprise around 40% of your energy needs for that day. This means 2 - 3 servings a day, covering approximately one quarter of your plate. This can be equated to any one of the following: one slice of bread, one cup of cooked rice, half a cup of grains or cereals, 300 grams (10 ounces) of milk or 200 grams (7 ounces) of plain yogurt.

At this point you might be worried that your diet is going to be highly restrictive. However, you will be glad to know that you can still enjoy a filling and satisfying meal if you fill half of your plate with what most experts refer to as "free foods."

These are the types of foods that are low in carbohydrate, fat, or protein content but still contain plenty of fiber, as well as essential vitamins and minerals. The following are recognized as 'free foods': grapefruit, passion fruit, lemons, rhubarb, pickles, mustard, chutney, spices and herbs, as well as all of the vegetables (except potatoes, sweet corn and sweet potatoes).

Anti-Diabetes Super Food

Nature has produced certain foods that you can consume to actually help you treat diabetes. One such powerful super food is bitter gourd or bitter melon. A lot of research has proven the effectiveness of bitter gourd in lowering blood glucose levels. The key is in the combination of steroidal saponin, peptides that are similar to insulin, and alkaloids. Furthermore, consuming bitter gourd helps boost the cells' intake of glucose, stimulate the pancreas to release insulin and boost the actions of insulin itself. Lastly, the natural chemicals in bitter gourd help to regulate cholesterol and triglyceride levels.

A lot of people do not like the taste of bitter gourd, which makes it a kind of bitter medicine for diabetes. However, it is advised that you include bitter gourd at least once a day in your meals to ensure that your diet is centered on fighting diabetes. To reduce the bitterness, you can do the following: wash the bitter gourd very well, as you will be eating the skin. Then, cut it in half across and then cut each piece into half, lengthwise. With a spoon, remove the core of the bitter gourd and scrape away much of the white meat. Slice the bitter gourd thinly. You can then soak it in salted water or pineapple juice to further reduce the bitterness. It is preferably eaten raw as a salad to help conserve its nutrients.

CHAPTER 5

Exercising With Diabetes

Time and time again, experts stress the importance of regular physical activity for both diabetics and non-diabetics. Research has, in fact, proven that diabetics who engage in exercise, follow their diet plan and take their medication properly enjoy normalized blood glucose, among other health benefits. Exercise also minimizes your need for insulin and other medications.

For safety reasons, a diabetic who has been living a sedentary lifestyle in the past needs to consult a doctor before following any regular exercise regimen. Talk to your doctor about the exercises that you need to avoid because of your diabetes. For example, if you have diabetic retinopathy you should avoid weight lifting, bouncing exercises and scuba diving or mountain climbing. If you have diabetic neuropathy you must not do any pounding exercises. For those who have kidney disease, exercises that will raise blood pressure for a long period of time should be avoided, such as long distance running.

At the start of the regimen, ensure that you are wearing comfortable workout clothes, including cotton socks and cushioned athletic shoes to minimize strain and reduce the risk of injuries. Drink water about 20 minutes before your workout, take small sips during, and gradually drink plenty of water afterward. It is advisable that you exercise with a friend who understands hypoglycemia to help you in case you experience it. Keep a piece of candy in your pocket in case you are feeling unwell during your workout.

Add variety to your workouts in order to avoid getting bored with them. After all, you will be exercising regularly for the rest of your life so why not make it fun? Choose a moderate exercise such as jogging to start. Ideally, moderate exercise should be performed for 30 to 45 minutes and at least 3 or 4 times each week. Medical and fitness experts recommend 150 minutes a week. Alternate your exercise regimen between cardiovascular exercises, resistance or strength training, and flexibility exercises to address the different needs of your body.

These are the types of exercise recommended for people with diabetes. They are also excellent for anyone who may be overweight and not used to exercising regularly. Best of all, you don't need special equipment for them, so you can get started right away.

Walking

Walking is excellent all-round exercise, and you don't need any special equipment, other than a comfortable pair of supportive shoes. This is particularly important for diabetics, since one of the complications of the condition is loss of feeling in the extremities, due to poor circulation. There are special shoes around which are designed with diabetics in mind, to offer extra support and cushioning. Ask your medical team about this.

Regular aerobic exercise such as walking helps to regulate the body's blood sugar levels, as well as making it easier for the body to use insulin effectively. These benefits are particularly important for diabetics, although they benefit everyone, as they help to keep internal inflammation under control. This is often linked with obesity and chronic health conditions such as obesity, auto-immune system diseases, heart disease and arthritis, among others.

Walking also raises 'good' HDL cholesterol levels, while simultaneously lowering the 'bad' LDL cholesterol, thus protecting against heart disease and stroke, both of which can be potentially fatal complications of diabetes.

If you can't fit in long walks, try to take several short walks each day. How long you walk for is not important. What really matters is that you walk fast enough to increase your heart rate to give your heart and lungs a good aerobic workout and burn calories to help you keep your weight at a healthy level, or lose any excess pounds.

Perhaps one of the overlooked benefits of walking is that it releases endorphins – the 'feel good' chemicals that help to alleviate stress. Stress produces hormonal imbalances in the body, and since diabetes does the same thing, it can mess around with the way you feel big time. Exercise helps to counteract that, so that you're less likely to feel stressed and depressed.

Swimming and water exercise

Swimming is excellent exercise for anyone suffering from a chronic health condition, since anyone, whatever their age, weight, state of health or fitness level can do it. It's also enjoyable, which means you are more likely to stick with it, so it's a more viable proposition for diabetics, who need regular exercise in their lives on a permanent basis. It's a social form of exercise too – you can go along with friends, children and grandchildren and have great fun while you do your body a big favor and give it a regular healthy dose of aerobic exercise.

The big plus with swimming is that it supports the entire weight of the body, so it's less stressful on the joints. That means that absolutely anyone can swim, whereas they might not be able to do other forms of exercise. And swimming works every major muscle group in the body, so it's a complete all over workout.

Another thing to consider is doing exercises in water. The resistance of the water increases the effects of the exercise as opposed to exercising on land, and it's also less tiring, as the water supports your weight and keeps you cooler. Exercising in water will also be more comfortable for people with diabetic neuropathy, so that's two good reasons for diabetics to head poolside.

Remember to let someone know you are diabetic, just in case of problems. Carry a healthy snack with you, in case you need to pack in some calories to avoid hypoglycemia. That's a consideration for all diabetics, so it's probably safer to go swimming with a buddy if you can. If that's not possible, remember to carry your medical ID. You have diabetes, and people need to know so that you can be safe while you swim.

Speaking of safety, if you swim in the ocean or the lake, wear swimming shoes to protect your feet from damage from stones and rocks. This is especially important if you suffer from diabetic neuropathy. When diabetics do any exercise, it's important to take safety into consideration, but it's particularly important when swimming, as the water increases the potential for problems.

Yoga

Yoga is an excellent all round exercise, and it's particularly helpful for diabetics because it's not just an exercise – practiced correctly, it's a lifestyle and a complete union of mind, body and spirit. Yoga practitioners are more in tune with their bodies and the way they work than other people, and this is ideal for diabetics, who need to know what their body is doing 24/7 if they are to stay fit and healthy.

Some poses stimulate the pancreas to produce more insulin, and yoga as a general discipline is known to promote organ health and improve and balance metabolic activity. Practitioners notice and improvement in their blood glucose levels, and also a drop in stress, which means there is less likelihood of stress hormones unsettling the body's delicate chemical balance and causing unwanted complications for diabetics.

Yoga is suitable for all ages and fitness levels. Since it benefits the endocrine and nervous systems, it is very effective in both the prevention and treatment of diabetes. However, it is advisable to go to a qualified teacher to learn how to do the poses properly, and also to warm up and cool down before and after the sessions. This is particularly important for diabetics, since all exercise carries a certain element of risk. Learning the correct way to do the poses and implement the right breathing techniques will keep your yoga sessions safe and beneficial.

The yoga diet is high in fiber and very healthy, and this too is perfect for diabetics, since it balances blood sugar levels and helps them to lose any excess weight. Also, one bonus with yoga is that you become more in tune with your body's needs, and over time, you'll naturally avoid any foods that make you feel sluggish or bloated, and gravitate to the foods that help you to feel healthy. In effect, your body polices itself, and reacts against processed foods and foods high in fats and sugars. Yoga should play a part in everyone's exercise routine – especially if they are diagnosed with diabetes.

Tai Chi

Tai chi is an ancient Chinese martial art which has been practiced for thousands of years. Anyone of any age or fitness level can practice tai chi. It's low impact exercise, and there is no pain associated with it. It's a great stress buster, and the slow, controlled, graceful movements improve the balance and boost the circulation. These are two big pluses for diabetics, who may have nerve damage through diabetic neuropathy. Because tai chi helps the body to relax, so that all the internal processes are able to proceed effectively, which makes for better health.

While it's not a great calorie burner, tai chi does improve the metabolic process by improving the circulation, so in an indirect way it can help with weight loss and maintenance. It also helps the immune system to work more effectively, so that internal inflammation is reduced. As this is responsible for obesity and many chronic illnesses, tai chi can prevent the development of certain chronic conditions, as well as helping in the management of diagnosed illnesses such as diabetes.

Like yoga, tai chi encourages a mind, body spirit union which puts people more in tune with their bodies, and this is very helpful in the management of diabetes. It's fun, and it's easy to do, since the movements are slow and controlled. In no time, you'll be doing them automatically, allowing your mind to relax and all life's stresses to loosen their grip on you.

Dancing

Dancing makes this list because it's aerobic exercise and it's fun, and if you enjoy something, you're more likely to stick with it long term. If you are diabetic, you need to exercise regularly for life, not just while you're trying to lose excess weight. Exercise is a vital component of diabetes management, and dancing can burn up to 150 calories in half an hour. So as well as being great fun, it will help you to keep your weight under control and thus avoid the complications that can arise from being overweight and diabetic.

Dancing is social exercise, so you'll meet new people and have fun, and that's important when you have a chronic condition. You want your life to be as normal as everyone else's, and dancing is something almost everyone does. As with other forms of exercise, make sure the people you are with know about your diabetes and what to do if you have a problem. You should also carry a healthy snack in case you need a calorie boost, and make sure to drink plenty of water to avoid becoming dehydrated.

While exercise is very important for diabetics, it is also vital to exercise safely and effectively. That means ensuring that instructors and people accompanying you to exercise sessions or on walks or swims know that you are diabetic, and also know what to do if you become ill during the session. Keep a healthy snack with you at all times, and drink plenty of water before, during and after your exercise session.

Aim for regular, moderate exercise. Rather than hitting it with a two and a half hour session once a week, it's better to do five 30 minute sessions spread through the week to keep the metabolism and the circulation functioning well. And before stating any exercise program, check with your medical team, in case there are any special considerations you need to consider.

Generally speaking though, exercise can only be good for people with diabetes, so don't let your condition hold you back from getting the healthy exercise you need to manage your health.

CHAPTER 6

Understanding Diabetic Neuropathy

Diabetic neuropathy has been mentioned several times during the course of this book, but most people don't really understand exactly what it is, and how it affects them if they have diabetes. Maybe it's time to discuss exactly what it is, what causes it and what you can do if you suffer from diabetic neuropathy as a complication of diabetes.

Put simply, diabetic neuropathy is nerve damage caused by various factors associated with diabetes. Smoking and excessive alcohol consumption can contribute to this nerve damage, as can metabolic factors and auto-immune system problems. Also, the longer you have had diabetes, the more likely you are to develop a diabetic neuropathy. Injuries can also cause nerve damage.

Around 60 – 70% of all diabetics have some form of neuropathy, and most of those will have been diabetic for at least 25 years, so time has a lot to do with it. If your blood sugar levels are not stable, that can contribute to it too. There are four types of diabetic neuropathy – peripheral, which affects the extremities and is the more common kind, autonomic, which affects the digestion, sexual response and bowel and bladder function, as well as affecting the heart and blood pressure, and lungs and eyes.

Proximal neuropathy mainly affects the hips, thighs and legs, while focal neuropathy can affect any nerves or groups of nerves in the body. Here is a more detailed examination of the four types of neuropathy.

Peripheral neuropathy

This is the most common form of neuropathy, affecting the legs, feet, hands and arms. It is more likely to affect the feet and legs ahead of the arms and hands. Symptoms may take a long time to develop, and it's likely your doctor will notice them before you do. These symptoms can include tingling or numbness in the extremities, sharp pains and cramps, problems with co-ordination and balance and either insensitivity or hypersensitivity to pain, temperature or touch.

Peripheral neuropathy can also affect the reflexes and weaken the muscles, leading to deformities and even amputation if the condition is not diagnosed and treated in a timely manner. By maintaining safe, steady blood glucose levels, you can protect your nerves from damage, so it's important to monitor these levels regularly.

Autonomic neuropathy

Although it is not so common as peripheral neuropathy, the autonomic version can do a lot of damage, since it can affect the organs of the body as well as various systems such as the respiratory system and digestive system. It can also compromise the mechanism by which the body recovers from a hypoglycemic attack. This could disrupt the body's natural warning system, so that you don't receive warnings of an imminent hypoglycemic episode. This can be very dangerous.

Autonomic neuropathy also affects the nerves of the heart and blood vessels, and can cause fluctuations in blood pressure, as well as affecting the heart's ability to self-regulate the heart beat as you take part in different activities. This can be potentially fatal.

The digestive system can be badly affected by the condition, with constipation or diarrhea being common, or even an alternation between the two. Also, there can be problems swallowing and digesting food, leading to bloating, nausea, loss of appetite and weight loss. If the nerves of the urinary tract are affected, there may be difficulty emptying the bladder, which could lead to infections and eventual incontinence, while sexual enjoyment may also be adversely affected for both men and women.

Autonomic neuropathy can also compromise the body's natural cooling system, preventing the sweat glands from functioning normally to cool down the body. The condition is very distressing, since it can affect numerous areas of the body, as well as the internal organs.

Proximal neuropathy

This affects the lower half of the body, including the legs, hips, thighs and buttocks, and often just affects one side of the body. It is more common in older diabetics, and there may be problems in rising from sitting to standing unassisted. The condition can be very painful, as well as causing muscle weakness. Recovery from proximal neuropathy can be protracted, and can cause significant problems with mobility.

Focal neuropathy

This is usually sudden onset, and particularly affects the nerves in the legs, head and torso. It can cause Bell's Palsy, double vision and severe chest and abdominal pains which may be confused with appendicitis or a heart attack, so it's particularly distressing, and also unpredictable. The only good thing about focal neuropathy is that it doesn't seem to cause lasting damage, and it will clear up eventually. While it lasts though, it can be very painful and distressing.

Treating neuropathy

The main treatment for all types of diabetic neuropathy is to bring the blood glucose levels back into the acceptable, safe range. This may intensify symptoms at first, but it is the single most important treatment. Pain relief may also be prescribed, along with anti-depressants and anticonvulsants. The use of antidepressants is more for relaxing the muscles than treating depression, since muscle relaxants can offer significant relief from nerve pain. Just trust your doctor to prescribe the most appropriate treatment for your neuropathy.

Acupuncture and magnetic therapy may also be used to help alleviate symptoms. There are a number of effective treatments available for diabetic neuropathy, and your doctor can help to decide the best course of treatment in your particular case.

Diabetic neuropathy is no joke. Left untreated, it can result in amputation. While it can be pretty devastating, diabetic neuropathy can also be prevented, if you know what you're doing. Keep a close eye on blood glucose levels, and try to bring them down to more stable levels as quickly as possible. Get to know your body, so you can spot a potentially difficult health situation before it happens.

Apply a little common sense. If your neuropathy causes blood pressure and circulation problems, move around slowly to minimize the symptoms. You should also take particular care of your feet, since foot problems are common in diabetic neuropathy, and can lead to amputation. Prevention is better than cure, so take real good care of your feet and legs.

Diabetic neuropathy is a distressing condition, but it is preventable and also treatable. Keep an eye on your blood glucose levels, and hopefully this will prevent the development of diabetic neuropathy. However, if the condition does manifest itself, work closely with your health care providers in order to apply the most up effective and up to date treatment options.

CHAPTER 7

Alcohol and Diabetes

Alcohol doesn't have to be totally off limits if you have diabetes, so you may be able to celebrate with an occasional drink on special occasions. However, alcohol can cause complications in people with diabetes, so you need to be aware of what alcohol can do, and what is a safe drinking level in your case. General guidelines are one unit of alcohol per day for women and two for men, and it's not advisable to save them up for a binge at the weekend, as this can play havoc with your blood glucose levels.

The effectiveness of some medications may be impaired by alcohol, so check with your doctor to ensure this is not so in your case. If the doctor says it's okay for you to drink, don't just dive in and drink everything in sight, because this could cause problems and complications with your diabetes.

You need to be aware of your blood glucose levels, and you should never drink on an empty stomach. It's not a good idea for anyone, but it's asking for trouble if you are diabetic. Alcohol can impact on the production and release of glucose by the liver, which means you could end up with dangerously low levels of blood glucose. The liver prioritizes tasks, and processing the alcohol is more important as far as the liver is concerned than producing glucose.

Blood sugar levels be affected for up to 24 hours after your last drink, so you need to closely monitor your glucose levels before, during and after drinking alcohol, otherwise you could end up with a hypoglycemic incident. The problem is, the symptoms of this are similar to the symptoms of excessive consumption of alcohol – dizziness, sleepiness and disorientation. Be sure to wear a medical ID, so that if you become ill, people will not just assume you are drunk, and will summon medical help. It's a good idea to check your blood glucose levels before bed when you've been drinking alcohol. If the levels are low, have a snack before you go to sleep.

Some alcoholic drinks are very high in sugar, so you should avoid these. Liqueurs such as Baileys and sweet wines can cause hypoglycemia, as can sugary mixers, so choose your drinks with care. Extra strong alcoholic drinks can also impact on blood glucose levels. It may be a good idea to make a long drink like a wine spritzer, or intersperse alcoholic drinks with water or diet soda to keep yourself hydrated.

You can mitigate the effects of alcohol on blood glucose by always having food with your drink. Even a couple of crackers is better than nothing, so always plan to eat something when you drink. It's all a question of considering the impact of the alcohol on your blood sugar levels, and doing what you can to avoid potential problems.

As for drink choices, go for dry wines or light beers, as they are lower in calories and alcohol than other alcoholic drinks. If you choose to drink spirits, make a long drink with a diet soda or sparkling water to dilute the alcohol and make the drink last for longer. Sip your drink rather than throwing it back, because you can't afford to have too much if you're going to keep your diabetes on an even keel.

If you are suffering from diabetic neuropathy, alcohol could exacerbate nerve damage, so it's best to avoid it altogether. Alcohol can intensify the pain, tingling and numbness associated with the condition, so it's really not worth drinking and risking more nerve damage.

Other conditions which may make it advisable to avoid alcohol are diabetic retinopathy (eye damage caused by diabetes), kidney disease and high blood pressure or high blood triglycerides.

Having read all this, you may decide that drinking alcohol is not worth the risk of potential problems and complications. That's a decision only you can make, with the help of your health care professionals. If you do decide to have the occasional drink, remember to monitor your glucose levels and inform the people you are with that you are diabetic, so they know to summon medical help if necessary.

CHAPTER 8

Looking After Your Heart With Diabetes

Taking care of your heart is important for everyone – it's the only heart you have, and if it fails, you die. However, since heart disease and stroke is responsible for around 65% of all deaths in people with diabetes, it's even more important to look after your heart. Diabetes increases the risk of heart disease and stroke by two to four times the normal risk for people who do not have diabetes, but the good news is, there is a lot that you can do to keep your heart and the blood vessels that are responsible for circulation healthy.

People with diabetes are more likely to develop heart disease because they also have conditions like high blood pressure and cholesterol and raised levels of triglycerides, as well as being overweight or obese. All of these are recognized risk factors for heart disease.

The first thing you need to do is examine your lifestyle. If you smoke, you should quit right now, as this increases the risk of heart disease and stroke, as well as raising blood pressure and cholesterol levels, both of which are significant risk factors for heart disease and stroke.

Aim to increase your activity levels so you are exercising for at least 30 minutes, five days a week. This is recommended as a management strategy for diabetes anyway, and it will help to keep your weight under control, which is another way to reduce the risk of developing heart disease as a complication of diabetes.

Educate yourself in heart healthy nutrition, because what you eat can help you to have a healthy heart. Go for lean meat, chicken and fish, and trim off all visible fat before eating. Cut down on salt, as this can elevate the blood pressure, and eat plenty of fiber, as it helps to keep blood cholesterol at healthy levels. Get fiber from whole grains, beans and pulses and fruit and vegetables.

Know your fats, and know what to go for and what to avoid. Trans fats, which are found mostly in shop bought bakery goods and other processed foods, raise cholesterol levels, which increases the risk of heart disease. Trans fats may also be labeled as 'hydrogenated oils.' Monounsaturated fats such as olive oil, peanut oil, avocado and almonds are much healthier, as are polyunsaturated fats like sunflower oil, corn oil and walnuts. Then there are the Omega-3 fatty acids found in oily fish such as tuna, salmon, mackerel and herring, which are particularly heart healthy.

The Mediterranean Diet is acknowledged as being one of the healthiest eating plans around, and it's especially good for heart health. It's also easy to follow, with no need for special foods or difficult to follow recipes. Another advantage of the

Mediterranean Diet is that it's not a diet as such – more a long term healthy eating plan, which is what you need.

Another excellent eating plan for a healthy heart is the DASH Diet (Dietary Approaches to Stop Hypertension). It's aimed at lowering blood pressure and cholesterol, and helping you to keep your weight at a healthy level, so it's ideal for diabetics who want to keep their hearts healthy. The next chapters will take a more detailed look at diets to avoid and healthy eating plans which are suitable for helping to avoid complications with diabetes, so if you are a little confused as to the best way to eat for heart health, worry no more. It's just as important to know which diets to steer clear of when you are diabetic, since some diets are more likely to cause potentially dangerous hypoglycemia than healthy weight loss.

Another way to protect your heart is to get enough exercise, to keep the circulation working well so that all of your internal organs are well supplied with blood and oxygen. Check out Chapter 5 for detailed information on exercising safely and effectively with diabetes, and remember to check on your blood sugar levels before, during and after exercise.

Also, have a snack handy if you need it, sip water to stay hydrated, and inform someone that you have diabetes, so that if you have a problem while exercising, they know what to do. Always wear your medical ID, so that you can get the help you need as quickly as possible in case of emergency. Although you can live a pretty normal life if you manage your diabetes well, you can never forget that you have it, because if you do, you're letting unwanted complications into your life.

Keeping your heart healthy with diabetes can actually be easier in some ways than it is for non-diabetics, since you need to be more in tune with how your body works in order to manage your condition effectively. It's well worth doing as well – the more proactive you are in avoiding the complications of diabetes, the healthier and happier you will be.

CHAPTER 9

Diet Plans People With Diabetes Should Avoid

People with diabetes have to be totally focused on the food they eat for several reasons. What you eat directly affects your blood glucose levels, and if they are erratic, there is more risk of diabetes-related complications such as neuropathies and heart disease developing. While these complications can be treated, prevention is always better than cure, and the best way to prevent complications with diabetes is to carefully control what you eat.

Another reason for focusing on food is to get the metabolism working efficiently and to lose any excess weight you may be carrying, since a sluggish metabolism and being overweight can exacerbate the symptoms of diabetes, as well as causing unwanted and potentially serious complications. It's worth remembering that around 65% of people who have diabetes die from heart disease or stroke, so following a heart healthy eating plan is a potential life-saver.

Most chronic conditions are made worse by internal inflammation, so it's a good idea to include as many anti-inflammatory foods in your diet as possible. This will also help with controlling any pain associated with diabetic neuropathy, since some foods are just as effective as anti-inflammatory drugs at relieving pain and reducing internal inflammation.

All this might sound a little confusing and scary, but there are a number of tailored eating plans which are ideal for diabetics, as they are low in fat and calories, but high in fiber, protein and antioxidants and vitamins. Importantly, these eating plans have been unanimously approved by medical experts all over the world, so you can be confident about using them to help manage your diabetes. In fact, you may wish to combine elements of several eating plans to suit your individual preferences and lifestyle.

A word of caution here – don't ever be tempted to follow an eating plan that is very restrictive, or eliminates entire food groups. As a diabetic, you need a healthy, balanced diet, with the right proportions of all the macronutrients such as proteins, carbohydrates and fats. A diet or eating plan that excludes the necessary nutrients could be positively dangerous. Also, very low calorie diets or meal replacement diets are not a good idea for diabetics. You should also avoid fad diets, or diets that restrict you to a small number of foods, even for a few days.

The Atkins and South Beach diets which are high in protein and low in carbohydrates can in some cases be suitable for diabetics, as they aim to produce ketosis in the body to encourage fat burning. Ketosis occurs when glucose stores are low, and the body has to burn fat for energy. However, for diabetics to safely follow this type of diet, they need to be closely supervised by their doctor, as their medications or insulin dose will need adjustment.

Many medical experts believe that the Atkins Diet is too low in carbohydrates to be safe for diabetics. There is also a real risk that diabetics may become hypoglycemic before they achieve ketosis, and that can be dangerous. In addition, the high levels of protein in the Atkins Diet can cause the kidneys to work overtime, and if you have kidney problems as a result of diabetes, following the Atkins Diet could exacerbate them.

The South Beach Diet is somewhat healthier, since it encourages you to eat healthy carbs, but the induction phase is too risky, as it is designed to induce ketosis. However, the maintenance stage is more suitable for diabetics.

Before beginning any new eating plan you should always check with your health care providers, in case the plan needs to be adapted to take your diabetes into consideration. Dieting is different when you have diabetes – never forget that.

Bear in mind that dieting carries the risk of hypoglycemia, and rapid weight loss diets significantly increase that risk, so that's another reason to run your intended eating plan past your doctor. High fiber diets that keep your blood glucose levels stable with the slow release of energy are less likely to cause hypoglycemia.

It's relatively easy to recognize a fad diet or a dangerous diet. They often ban or promote a particular food or food group at the expense of others, when a healthy diet should consist of foods from all food groups, in healthy proportions. And if a diet suggests that a particular food can mess around with the natural body chemistry, give it a wide berth, because your body knows best in that department. It's a wonderful, complex machine, and it's been around in its present form for a hell of a lot longer than the fad diets that try to sell you an impossible ideal.

The foolproof way to check whether a particular diet is a good fit with diabetes is to run it past your doctor. If he's not happy, you shouldn't be either. And if a diet is really healthy for diabetics, it will be endorsed by your national Diabetic Association, so that's a further safety check. Don't fall for the hype – check it out with the people who are best qualified to advise you.

In summary, all diets are not necessarily healthy ways for diabetics to lose weight. Diets that restrict certain foods or food groups, or do not provide enough carbohydrates are not good choices, nor are very high protein diets which could cause kidney problems in diabetics. Very low calorie diets are also a bad idea, since diabetics need a certain amount of calories to keep blood sugar levels stable, otherwise there is a real risk of a hypoglycemic incident. All weight loss diets carry this risk, particularly rapid weight loss diets, so it's important to check with your health care practitioners before embarking on any weight loss diet.

CHAPTER 10

Healthy Eating Plans For People With Diabetes

As discussed in Chapter 9, some eating plans and diets are just not suitable for people with diabetes. In fact, they can be positively dangerous, and cause more problems than they solve. So although it's very important to eat healthily with diabetes, you also need to be aware of the possible pitfalls. Perhaps the most important point to remember is that any weight loss diet has the potential to trigger hypoglycemia.

Diets advertised as 'fast weight loss' or very low calorie diets are particularly likely to do this, so it may be a better idea to follow a healthy eating plan which gives you all the nutrients you need from all the major food groups. Combined with the right amount of exercise, you should lose any excess pounds slowly and safely.

The problem with diets is that they smack of the temporary. You 'go on' a diet, and when you've lost the weight you need to lose you 'come off' the diet. Hopefully you'll keep up with the good habits that helped you to lose the weight, and you'll be able to keep it off. Chances are though that you won't, and the pounds will creep back on, with maybe a few extras to keep them company. Then you 'go on' the diet again, and so it continues.

You're now entered into a cycle of yo-yo dieting, and that's not good news for someone with diabetes. Yo-yo dieting plays havoc with your blood glucose levels – it's far better to formulate a healthy eating plan that ticks all the boxes for people with diabetes. And if the thought of formulating a healthy eating plan scares you, there are a number out there that can do it for you, and what's more, medical professionals and nutritionists endorse them as being among the healthiest diets for anyone. That's because they're full of nutrients and antioxidants, and low on calories and fats. These, then, are some of the healthiest long term eating plans for people with diabetes.

The Mediterranean Diet

The Mediterranean Diet is not a diet as such, rather it's a healthy way of eating adopted by the countries in the Mediterranean region. It's based around healthy ingredients such as fruit and vegetables, and lean proteins like fish, eggs and poultry. The diet is pretty much devoid of processed food, and most meals are cooked from scratch with natural, in season ingredients. If a Mediterranean wife doesn't recognize something as food, she won't cook with it.

Fat in the Mediterranean Diet is based mainly around olive oil, which is a healthy, monounsaturated fat which is known to be beneficial for the heart. The Mediterranean Diet is also light on pastry and baked goods, so it's a low fat, low calorie way of eating.

Most of the fruits and vegetables used in the Mediterranean Diet are brightly colored – peppers, tomatoes, berries, leafy greens, sweet potatoes, cantaloupe melons and citrus fruits all make an appearance. Brightly colored fruits and vegetables are known to be high in vitamin content and antioxidants. For someone with diabetes, that's good news, as these foods support the immune system and fight internal inflammation, which is a common feature of diabetes and other chronic conditions.

The Mediterranean Diet is high in fiber, because fruit and vegetables feature significantly. Fiber helps you to stay fuller for longer, which is great if you are trying to lose a few pounds to make your diabetes more manageable. It also helps to regulate blood sugar levels, since it releases energy steadily, thus avoiding sugar spikes. And fiber helps to keep the heart healthy. Since around 65% of people with diabetes die from heart disease or stroke, that's a big plus point.

Anti-inflammatory diet

Inflammation occurs when there is a perceived threat to the health and well being. It's an automatic response from the immune system, and it can be external or internal. Internal inflammation is responsible for a number of health issues, including diabetes. As internal inflammation affects the organs, it's potentially dangerous, and the main cause of internal inflammation is diet. Literally, you are what you eat, so if you have diabetes, maybe you need to examine your eating habits and make some changes.

Anti-inflammatory diets are closely based on the Mediterranean Diet, with the emphasis on foods with anti-inflammatory properties. That's pretty much all the brightly colored fruits and vegetables, along with oily fish and whole grains. Google 'Anti-inflammatory foods' for a comprehensive list, and include as many of them as you can into your diet.

Some foods are so high in anti-inflammatory properties they can do the work of anti-inflammatory drugs, but without the side effects, so if you have a medical history which precludes the use of anti-inflammatory medication, this can be especially beneficial for you. If you suffer from hypertension or heart disease – which very often accompanies diabetes – or if there is a family history of those conditions, it could be dangerous for you to take anti-inflammatory medication. Some of these drugs – particularly COX enzyme inhibitors – can cause a stroke, so although they are very effective at dealing with internal inflammation, the cure could very well be worse than the disease.

Recent research suggests that some fruits can work just as well as COX inhibitors, and strawberries are at the top of the list. A bowl of strawberries 3 or 4 times a week is as effective against internal inflammation as the strongest COX inhibitors, without the unwelcome side effects. And isn't it so much nicer to get your medication from something you enjoy?

Other great anti-inflammatory foods are all kinds of berries and brightly colored fruits, so think cherries, blueberries, cantaloupe and watermelons. It's the same with vegetables, so go for peppers, sweet potatoes, carrots and green leafy vegetables. The great thing about an anti-inflammatory diet is that it's really flexible, so you can go with the foods you love.

It may take a while to see results, but after a few weeks, you'll probably notice that you have more energy, and you may even lose a few pounds in weight. Another plus is that the reduction in inflammation will bring a corresponding reduction in pain, so if you're troubled with diabetic neuropathy, you should notice a lessening of pain in the nerve endings. Also, any other niggling aches and pains should clear up or become more manageable.

DASH (Dietary Approaches to Stop Hypertension) diet

As has been previously mentioned, heart disease and stroke account for around 65% of deaths in people with diabetes. Hypertension – elevated blood pressure – increases the risk of heart disease and stroke considerably. In fact, monitoring of blood pressure is one of the most important elements of the care plan for diabetics.

The DASH diet is aimed at reducing blood pressure and cholesterol levels, and is therefore concentrated on high fiber, low fat and low sodium eating, with healthy fats such as olive oil, and Omega-3 fatty acids from oily fish such as salmon, tuna and mackerel.

There's big emphasis on fruit and vegetables and lean protein from poultry, eggs, fish, pulses and beans. Processed foods and pastry products do not feature in this eating plan. Although the DASH diet is not specifically a weight reduction diet, you will find that you lose any excess weight as a result of following it, since, like the Mediterranean Diet, it focuses on fruit, vegetables and whole foods, which are generally low in calories and fat, and also help to boost the metabolism.

Another feature of the DASH diet is healthy fats in the form of olive oil and other monounsaturated fats. Everyone needs some fat for healthy body function, but animal-based saturated fats are the ones that clog the arteries. The DASH diet – and indeed all diets that are suitable for diabetics – concentrates on heart healthy fats.

The right diet for diabetes management is the key to feeling fit and healthy with diabetes and keeping complications to a minimum. If you eat right, you reduce the risk of diabetes-related complications such as neuropathies and heart disease. Also, the right diet will reduce internal inflammation, help you to lose excess weight and keep the metabolism functioning efficiently. In many cases, the right diet is all that is needed to keep diabetes under control. Not everyone requires insulin or medication, so it's worth taking the time to find the right diet for you.

Work with your doctor and nutritionist on this, because sometimes there are absorption problems with vitamins, due to the hormonal changes brought about by diabetes. It may be that you need to supplement your diet with extra vitamins and minerals. However, you should not do this without checking with your doctor first, as some supplements may impair the effects of any medication you are taking.

Finding the right eating plan with diabetes may take a little time, but by doing your own research, and working with your care providers, you will find a plan that works for you. It may need some adaptation to suit your individual needs, since diabetes affects different people in different ways.

CHAPTER 10

Avoiding Diabetes Complications

In the previous chapters, various complications of diabetes have been mentioned. Clearly, complications are something you'll wish to avoid, since they can have serious repercussions. Diabetic neuropathies can lead to amputations or blindness if not treated in a timely manner. Also, people with diabetes are more susceptible to heart disease. So it makes sense to avoid these complications if at all possible, since they can be life-limiting and even life-threatening. Here are some of the best ways of avoiding diabetes complications, so that you can enjoy a happy, active and healthy life, despite diabetes.

Manage, manage, manage

The most important thing you can do in order to avoid complications is to manage your diabetes actively, all the time. This really can't be stressed enough. Management means learning all you can about diabetes, and in particular how it affects you, because everybody's diabetes journey is different, although there are a number of common factors that apply to everyone with diabetes.

Sign up to respected websites and national associations, so you get news on the latest research developments and treatments, and a steady stream of hints and tips about managing diabetes actively and successfully. If there's a forum, join it, because everyone there has experienced what you are going through, and they can help with your queries. At the very least, you will get support from people who know what it's like to live with diabetes.

If there's a local support group, go along and make friends. Diabetes management is a lifetime commitment, and sometimes you can feel isolated and alone with your condition. Meeting others in the same situation will provide support and motivate you to keep managing.

Make healthy eating and regular exercise your main priorities, and learn how to manage your blood glucose levels. Monitor these closely, and ask your doctor for advice on regulating them. Erratic blood sugar levels are known to contribute to the most serious diabetic complications, so it's important that you know how to check them and how to bring them back under control.

Make friends with your medical team, and don't be afraid to ask for advice and help when you need it. They are the experts, and they would much rather answer your questions, even if they seem silly to you, than have to deal with the consequences of diabetic complications.

Swear off smoking

Smoking is bad news for your health, but it's even worse news for diabetics. If you're a smoker, you should quit if you are diagnosed with diabetes. Smoking increases your chance of diabetic complications, and some of them can be life-threatening, or at least life limiting.

Blood flow to the extremities can be restricted, and that can exacerbate the effects of diabetic neuropathies. In the worst case scenario, you may have to undergo amputations as a result of infections and ulcers in the legs and feet.

Smoking can also cause eye damage, which may eventually lead to blindness, and nerve damage and kidney damage is much more likely if you are a smoker. Smokers are also more at risk of heart disease and strokes. When you remember that 65% of deaths among diabetics are caused by heart attacks and strokes, you have to wonder why anyone with diabetes would choose to smoke.

If you are having difficulty kicking the nicotine habit, ask your medical team what help is available to you. You really need to quit, and quit sooner rather than later.

Watch blood pressure and cholesterol levels

Diabetes damages the blood vessels, and so does hypertension, or high blood pressure. While hypertension is a concern for everyone, it's particularly dangerous for diabetics, since the effects are magnified. It's the same with high levels of blood cholesterol. It's bad enough for anyone, but it's much worse for diabetics.

A healthy diet and regular exercise will go a long way to keeping blood pressure and cholesterol at healthy levels. However, you may need help from prescription medication, too. Get a home blood pressure monitor so you can keep a close eye on your blood pressure. Often, there are no symptoms until you have serious problems, so it's important to make regular checks and seek medical help if necessary. Your doctor will advise as to what is a healthy blood pressure reading for you. If it rises above that and stays elevated, consult your doctor as soon as possible.

Get regular check ups

Nobody likes to feel as if they are living at the medical center or hospital, but when you have diabetes, you need regular scheduled physical checks and eye examinations, to ensure that any complications are detected and treated as soon as possible.

Ideally, you should get two or three general physical checks each year, and get your eyes examined as often as your ophthalmologist recommends. This is likely to be at least once a year, so that they can pick up and treat signs of retinal damage, glaucoma or cataracts. Blindness is a real risk with diabetes – regular eye examinations can avoid that.

Physical check-ups involve running through your diet plan and exercise routine, checking your weight and investigating for any indicators of complications, such as nerve damage or kidney malfunction. Your doctor will also check for early signs of heart disease. The sooner diabetic complications are identified, the more chance there is of successful treatment and avoiding permanent damage.

Check if you need vaccinations

If you are diabetic, it's likely that high blood sugar levels have compromised your immune system, and it isn't working as effectively as it should. Your doctor may feel that you need certain vaccinations to keep you healthy and avoid complications. In particular, he may recommend flu and pneumonia shots in the fall. Hepatitis B vaccination is also recommended for diabetic adults younger than 60. Your doctor will know which vaccines are appropriate in your case, so be sure to check with him.

Health conditions such as flu and pneumonia can cause extra problems for diabetics, so if your doctor advises you to have shots, trust his judgment.

Look after your feet

Foot problems can be a real concern for diabetics. That's because high blood glucose can cause issues with blood flow, leading to infections and nerve damage, as well as tingling, numbness and pain. Keep feet clean and well moisturized, and be sure to dry thoroughly after showering and bathing. Dry skin can be a problem, but don't use moisturizer between the toes, as this could be a breeding ground for bacteria and infection.

Shoes made from natural fabrics such as leather, which allow the feet to breathe and offer support, are more suited for diabetics.

Make sure your feet are comfortable at all times, and if you have a sore spot or blister that doesn't heal within a few days, consult your doctor. Foot problems due to diabetes can lead to amputation if not dealt with promptly, so always be aware of anything that may require treatment.

Avoid stress

Stress can be harmful to health for anyone. While a little stress is healthy, too much can be positively dangerous, especially for diabetics. When the body is stressed, it produces hormones to deal with the situation – it's a throwback to the old 'fight or flight' mechanism of hunter-gatherer days. These hormones can seriously interfere with insulin production, and that can cause complications in the care and management of your diabetes.

There's a natural tendency to try to carry on as normal, despite your diabetes. It's almost as if you have something to prove to others, but in fact, this is the worst thing you can do. Diabetics are more prone to heart disease and stroke, and excessive stress can contribute to these conditions. Therefore part of your diabetes management should concentrate on stress management.

Learn to say No, and learn to prioritize. Some things are more important than others, so learn to sort out what can wait and what needs to be attended to right away. Nobody is indispensible – remember that, and don't take on more than you can reasonably manage.

Exercise can also help with stress management, as it releases 'feel good' hormones into the body. If you can't face the gym, get out swimming or walking with friends, or go to a dance. All exercise is good, so if you're feeling stressed, try it. Company is important if you're using exercise as a stress buster. It's very easy – and perfectly understandable - to feel sad and alone with your diabetes. Get out and have some fun with friends.

If you have problems relaxing and resting, try a yoga class, or learn some relaxation techniques so you can switch off from the day's concerns and just chill out. And make sure you get enough restful sleep. The body repairs and renews itself as you sleep, so it's important to get the rest you need, especially since diabetes can cause fatigue.

Write stuff down

This may seem obvious, but when you're managing diabetes, it's easy to just get into a habit of doing things in a particular way, then automatically adjusting, depending on the numbers. However, your doctor will want to look back at events over the period since he last saw you, and the best way for him to be able to do that is to look back over a written record, or for you to update him from notes on what's been happening since your last appointment.

It's not necessarily just the obvious stuff you need to record either. If you've had a particularly good day or bad day, write that down too, because you may be able to see a pattern emerging. Maybe certain foods make you feel better or worse, or maybe you need to step up or scale down your activity level. Get into the habit of keeping a diabetes journal, and recording stuff that strikes you as significant at the time, because by the time you go for your next appointment, you'll have forgotten all about it.

Always keep a list of your medications, whether over the counter or prescribed. If you need emergency treatment from someone who is not part of your regular care team, that's one of the first things they'll want to know. If you start to take a new drug, write down how you feel in the first few days, to pinpoint any side effects as they happen.

The most important thing is to stay positive with your diabetes management. Diabetes does not define you – it's just something you have to live with and cope with on a daily basis. In fact, most people with diabetes live and eat more healthily than other people. Being diagnosed with diabetes isn't the end of your world – it's merely a new phase on your journey through life, and one which you have more control over than you may realize.

CHAPTER 11

Misconceptions About Diabetes

Lots of people think they know all about diabetes, whether they are diagnosed with the condition or not. The fact is, there are still a lot of misconceptions flying around, and you need to be aware of them if you are to successfully manage your condition and live a healthy live with diabetes. Most of these misconceptions revolve around eating, and they can be summarized pretty briefly.

You do not need to eat specially made diabetic foods. These tend to be highly processed, and while they may be low in sugar and fat, they may not be as nutritious as natural whole foods. If you are following a healthy eating plan recommended by your care team or a national diabetic association, you don't need special foods. It's cheaper and healthier to just follow your plan.

You don't need to cut carbohydrates and sugar from your diet either. Complex carbs are high in fiber and can help you feel fuller for longer, which is great if you're trying to lose a few pounds. Fiber protects the heart from damage and disease as well.

Just because you have diabetes, it doesn't mean you can never have sweets or chocolate ever again. Any foods are fine in healthy amounts. Sweets and chocolate, like alcohol, should be an occasional treat rather than a major part of your diet. That goes for pretty much everyone, not just diabetics.

Some people say that diabetes is not a serious illness. Of itself, and properly managed, it is not. However, a diagnosis of diabetes places you at more risk of serious complications such as heart disease and stroke, which account for around one in three deaths among diabetics. Treat diabetes with respect, learn as much as you can about it and manage it well. If you can do all that, you can enjoy a long, healthy and happy life with diabetes. It's all about knowledge, so don't fall for the common misconceptions.

Conclusion

Diabetes can be managed and treated effectively, although the process of doing so requires knowledge, discipline, patience and passion. Your health and happiness does not have to drop along with your insulin and blood glucose levels. In fact, you can make your life even better if you learn as much as you can about how your body functions as a diabetic and follow a healthy lifestyle suitable for diabetics.

Most of the successful management of diabetes relies on the right food choices, and getting enough exercise. Diabetes is a long term condition which you will have to deal with for the rest of your life, but you can lead a full and active life when you are armed with the knowledge you need to understand and manage your condition.

Hypoglycemia is an ever present concern for diabetics. That's when the blood sugar levels drop dangerously low, and weight loss diets and too much exercise can cause a hypoglycemic incident. In fact, just about everything about diabetes revolves around blood glucose levels, so it's important that you understand how to keep these levels stable.

Diabetes in itself is not necessarily life-threatening, but there can be complications as a result of the condition and again, most of these complications can be attributed to fluctuating blood glucose levels, which can cause a lot of stress to the system. Most of the complications associated with diabetes – including diabetic neuropathies, retinal neuropathy, heart disease, high blood pressure and high cholesterol – can be prevented or controlled by keeping blood glucose levels within the healthy range.

Knowledge is power, so make sure you learn as much as possible about the treatment and management of diabetes, particularly how it affects you as an individual, because every diabetes journey is unique. What works for your friend or neighbor may not necessarily be the right thing for you.

Make friends with and make use of your health care providers, because they can help you to manage your condition effectively. They have seen all the complications and permutations, and they know how to address your concerns and help you through the bad spells and the down times. No matter how well you manage your diabetes, there will be times when nothing seems to go right, and you feel unwell, afraid and alone. The support of your family and your medical team will help you through those times.

Always wear your medical ID, and make sure that people you work with and socialize with know that you are diabetic, and what to do should you become ill. It's particularly important to notify the instructor if you attend an exercise class or the gym, so that they can take appropriate action to get you the treatment you need as quickly as possible should you have problems.

Above all, live your life as you want to, but always remember that you have diabetes and that there are adjustments you will need to make to your lifestyle if you are to stay fit and well. Treating and managing your diabetes will enable you to achieve the fit body and healthy lifestyle that everyone wants, whether or not they are diabetic. With the help of the tips and strategies in this book, you can start changing your life for the better right now.